Eating Clean But Keep It Lean

Weight Loss Clinic Secrets and Recipes – Brown Bag Lunches

Healthy Cooking made easy with American and European (metric and imperial) measures. Calorie, Fat, Protein and Carb calculations for every recipe

Cook and eat at home or brown bag it for lunch.

Maia Lloyd

Three Peas Publishing

First Edition

"Eating Clean But Keep It Lean" Series

DISCLAIMER

Introduction

You want to be healthy <u>and</u> lean…

I can help you with Eating Clean But Keep It Lean recipes

Welcome to the best brown bag lunch you have yet to eat.

The best because the food looks appetising and tastes great.

The really great thing is that this food is part of **the solution, not the problem, to getting and staying lean.** Plus, you won't be sacrificing your long term health in the desire to fit into your skinny jeans.

What you will gain from this book:

1. The **knowledge to make your clean eating and weight loss efforts a success, based on my expertise as a nutritionist with five weight loss clinics** in London;
2. **Simple, delicious recipes that are tried and tested in my weight loss clinics** to help you get and stay lean;
3. **Everyday ingredients, no faddy things you have never heard of**; and
4. **Encouragement to commit to this supportive, sustainable way of eating**. No three juices a day and starvation. Real, nutritious food to help you look great, prevent disease and age well.

It works for my clients and it can work for you.

Why my brown bag lunches are better

Let's start with what my lunch recipes <u>do not contain</u>: There are no mass-manufactured crisp breads, no factory-produced low fat fruit yoghurts and no awful polystyrene rice cakes. That is traditional brown bag lunch diet food – dull, artificial and joyless. If you want that kind of brown bag lunch food, you need read a different recipe book. The one you're looking for is called *"Eat Processed Diet Punishment Junk For Lunch: For Low Energy and Poor Results"*.

Since you are reading this, I think it is safe to assume that you are a bit more aspirational than that.

The recipes in this book include:

- Home-made pitta pockets with Thai-style Crayfish and Cucumber
- Turkey and Cranberry on Spelt and Seed Loaf sandwich
- Marakesh Chicken Salad on Buckwheat Bread
- Prawn Cocktail Wrap
- Middle Eastern Chickpea, Coconut and Spinach Lunchpot
- Provencal Tuna and Ratatouille Lunchpot
- Sweet and Sour Pork Lunchpot

That sound like a good lunch, don't you think?

This series is called "Eating Clean But Keep It Lean" because my approach is clean eating (which I will explain later on, if you are unclear). I focus on dropping weight as part of a clean diet so I will support your healthy aims and help you identify the elements of clean eating that may be holding your weight loss back.

My recipes are deliberately simple so you can use them every day. No long ingredients lists or complicated food prep.

In the back of your mind may be the idea that the choice is between two poles: healthy at one end and super lean at the other.

Healthy is a priority because you have to live in your body and everything from how you feel, to your ability to perform at work or in the sport you love or to run around after your children, to the quality of retirement you have is dependent on your health.

But, you also want to get lean and to do this you may believe that you have to restrict calories severely, eat horrible food or even resort to diet drugs or the body builder's favourite, human growth hormone (illegal, by the way, unless you are an under growth child and the doctor prescribes it) to shed the fat.

I am here to say that this polarity is simply wrong. You can have a super-healthy and clean diet with lots of variety and no obssessing about calories and still get and stay super lean.

But first..

Why listen to me?

Well, I am a nutritionist with five specialist weight loss clinics.

I help clients to lose weight and keep it off.

If someone pays to come and see me, they expect results. I often have clients for whom I am the last resort: They have tried to go it alone, they have tried group programmes, they may even have tried various therapies. They have probably struggled with their weight for years. Some also have a history of addictions or recreational drug use which, in my experience can cause long term low grade depression or be part of a compulsive streak, both of which can result in over-eating.

I do have clients for whom weight is only a very recent issue. Some lucky women don't have to worry about their weight in their teens, twenties or even thirties. But as menopause approaches so their appetite increases, driven by hormonal changes. Suddenly, they can't get into any of their clothes.

Others have worked so hard to be slim, over-exercising or ruthlessly sticking to 1000 calories a day, that it has affected their overall well being. I now have clients who, thanks to the wonders of technology, are ruled by their FitBits, the wrist bands that measure the number of steps you do a day and even the quality of your sleep. Fitbiters can become totally fixated on inputting calorie details and reading their results so that it becomes an obsession.

At the extreme end of this scale are those who go on liquid food replacement diets aka Very Low Calorie Diets (VLCDs).

Why very low calorie diets don't work

I have clients who have been on medically-mandated extreme weight loss diets. These are sometimes recommended by doctors for those whose weight is contributing to a life-threatening illness or condition such as liver disease, diabetes, high blood pressure and/or high cholesterol. Those who want to have gastric bypass surgery are sometimes told they need to get their weight down beforehand. The reason is anaesthetic is often dangerous if you are severely overweight.

And, certainly swapping to a VCLD for a few weeks can have dramatic effects. Without the tempation of real food around, some people lose a lot of weight, 14 pound/ 5 kilos or more a month by just having three shakes a day. But and it's a very big but, this weight loss is rarely sustainable. At some point you are going to need to go back to 'normal' food and at this point it can feel like the floodgates opening. The extreme body hunger that can result from VCLDs means that many people start eating and just can't stop.

The speed at which someone loses weight on a VLCD can also be a problem as we know that when you crash diet, you lose muscle as well as fat. If taken to extremes, this sort of diet can actually cause wasting in the muscles of your heart, causing a heart attack. More prosaically, loss of muscle causes a slow down in your metabolic rate so that when you do go back to eating, you gain weight much more easily. It is not the imagination of those failed VLCDers to think that post diet they only have to look at a doughnut to gain a pound. It is actually true.

The third problem is that VLCDs do not retrain you to enjoy healthy food, eat in balance, control your portion size or eat mindfully. All of these are important skills for keeping the weight off. VLCDs are about punishing yourself for the sins (over-eating) of the past.

One other version of the VLCD that I see at my clinics is that adopted by body builders.

Why eating like a bodybuilder doesn't work

There are many things that body builders get right. True bod builders strive for physical balance to create unity and symmetry in their physiques. However, they are not nutritionists. They are hyper-competitive and it is all about competition.

It is not fantasy to suggest that if you offered to inject a body builder with a secret drug which would give them 5% body fat overnight, most would say yes without asking any more questions.

There are exceptions to this and some body builders do develop some expertise in nutrition, but the majority do not. They take their nutritional advice from other body builders and just eat what their herd eats.

So what are the good things that body builders eat? A lot lean chicken and tuna, antioxidant-packed sweet potato and high protein boiled eggs, milk and yoghurt. Not so good are the post work out sugary drink and pre-work-out coffee (high in caffeine, which distrupts blood sugar).

The real problem with the bodybuilder diet is it is so restrictive. The proof of how grim it is lies in what happens in the 'off season' when they don't compete. As they know they won't be judged competitively on their physique, many loosen the nutritional reins and rebound eat.

In the same way a dieter who falls off their diet immediately stuffs themselves on all the things they have not been allowed to eat, so many bodybuilders over-eat in off season The result is they can gain a lot of weight. Logic suggests that if their on season diet was a bit more interesting, they wouldn't gain the weight in the off season?

Once they have gained the weight, they have to take it off again and this means both working out really, really hard, and cutting calories right back. This combination is incredibly punishing mentally and physically.

As an example of this, a new client came to see me at one of my clinics. He was a physique model and, to me at least, he looked amazing. So what did he want to see me about? The issue was the cost he was paying to be lean. He was exhausted most of the time and actually had a mid afternoon nap. This client was 22 years old! Why was he sleeping? His energy problems were undoubtedly caused by what he was eating .

Breakfast was malted loaf, a semi-sweet processed bread. The bread was a highly refined wheat flour loaf with added dried fruit for sweetness. This was a cocktail of sucrose and fructose with high fructose corn syrup added for good measure. This cocktail guaranteed him a sugar rush immediately after he had eaten, followed by an energy crash within 90 minutes. He felt dreadful mid morning.

Lunch was the same every day – a grey looking piece of broiled chicken breast and a large serving of white rice. No vegetables, no salad. It was low in nutrients and healthy fats and off the scale in sugar thanks to that white rice. And dinner was identical – broiled chicken and white rice. The boredom must have been unbelievable.

This is in my experience a pretty typical body builder diet. He was using the sugar to power his work out and the lean protein to build muscle, but he had nothing else to make the rest of this body work well. Low essential fats meant unstable or low mood and poor skin. A lack of antioxidants from the vegetables and fruit he wasn't eating was damaging his immune system, making him more liable to infection and problems associated with over-training.

The narrowness of his diet meant he was also likely to be depleted of other key minerals such as iron, zinc and magnesium, contributing to his feelings of tiredness and anxiety. Finally, a critical lack of fibre was putting him at risk of developing digestive problems and high cholesterol.

The most important reason NOT to adopt a diet like this is how it makes you feel, though. Even leaving aside the fact that your brain and hormonal systems cannot work effectively without healthy omega 3 fats , the massively restrictive nature of this sort of diet makes it impossible to be part of the world. You can't go out to eat, you can't eat at friends houses. You probably have to eat alone even if you're at home with your family.

As for my bodybuilder client, we worked together to agree an eating plan which he was confident would not raise his body fat but I was confident would also give him energy to do more than sleep. We upped his vegetables (with a lot of enouragement, he did not like vegetables, he said), and swapped the white rice for brown to increase fibre. We increased the variety of his meals.

Key to all of this was creating a healthy, brown bag lunch to stabilise his blood sugar so that reactive hypoglycaemia didn't make him sleepy in the afternoon. Out went broiled chicken and white rice. In came mexican bean dip with vegetables, lean coleslaw and sweet and sour pork (all recipes in this book). I am pleased to say he came second in his weight class at his national physique championships. So, clearly his ripped state was maintained but his mood and energy levels were massively improved.

So, you're heard a bit of what not to do, now let's talk about how you can lose weight get lean and be healthy. Let's start with the basics of clean eating

What is clean eating?

Eating clean means eating whole foods, in as natural a state as possible. It can include raw foods or vegetarian or vegan dishes. But equally, organic meat and fish can sit within the clean eating definition, if prepared freshly and sourced well.

The point is: clean eating is about showing respect for your body. It can be a way for those who have yo-yo dieted to stop calorie counting, then bingeing and then punishing themselves, to take a more positive approach to looking after their bodies.

If you stop obessively counting calories and studying your bottom in the mirror and instead adopt clean eating as a way to be healthy, you will not only be doing great things for your body but for your mind too.

Traditional diet foods tend to be highly processed and loaded with unhealthy ingredients like sweeteners. Low fat yoghurts and even humous has added sugar. The list of e numbers on the pack of a diet meal is scary.

Clean eating helps you to nourish your body and your mind, making you feel good about your efforts.

A word about sugar

While clean eating is the basis of my clinics' programmes, I do think that some versions out there are incredibly high in sugar. If you are concerned about your weight or just your health, tipping a shed load of sugar, whether it's called honey, brown rice syrup or coconut nectar, into your diet is not a good idea.

A high sugar diet puts you at risk of developing Type 2 diabetes and is a risk factor for many other serious health problems including cancer.

But, you say, I thought clean eating was low in sugar. Yes, it's low in processed sugars such as glucose and sucrose, but there are other 'natural' sugars out there from sources such as fruits, dried fruits, honey etc. you need to watch. Why? Because all sugars, natural or not, disrupt your blood sugar and therefore your energy levels, hormone balance and your mood. They also add excess calories, preventing your body getting lean.

I'm not suggesting you never eat an apple again. But I do recommend that you minimise certain 'natural' sugars, in addition to normal sucrose and high fructose corn syrup (which you won't be eating as junk food is off the menu anyway). These extra 'natural sugars to minimise are:

Fructose – from fruit;

Maple syrup – has healthy minerals but is still sugar;

Brown rice syrup – think of it as syrup dressed up as healthy. Eveything is relative I suppose and compared to golden syrup it is but not on my nutritional programmes;

Coconut sugar/nectar – it may be called "nectar" but it still counts as sugar;

Grape juice/apple juice – a common sweetener added to health store snacks;

Dates – most 'healthy' cookies and brownies are sweetened with these. Yes, they have useful minerals, but they are very high in sugar;

Agave syrup – this is a tricky one. It's a syrup processed from cacti. The jury is still out on how this affects your body. It may process in your body like sugar. Some of my clients also find that it affects their mood just like sugar. So take care with agave. See how you feel emotionally a few hours after eating it. Even if you feel fine, do not go overboard with agave; and

Stevia and xylitol – Less of a concern as they are both derived from natural sources and have both been shown not to affect blood sugar, but that doesn't mean you can use a ladle with them. Xylitol, if eaten to excess, can also cause stomach discomfort.

I use some fruit, Stevia and agave, but in moderation. Remember there no such things as a free lunch even with a Eating Clean But Keep It Lean lunch. If it tastes sweet it is a sourceof sugar, however supposedly healthy.

How to eat clean, lean and balanced

To balance the natural sugars in the clean eating staples of fruits and vegetables, it's really important to include proteins and fats too. Proteins help stabilise your blood sugar, preventing the roller-coaster ride that can cause bingeing. Fats stop your stomach emptying so you feel full.

The easiest way to stay clean but also balanced is to make sure every meal and snack includes carbs, proteins and fats together. If you want to do a juice, add some yoghurt for protein and some Chia seeds for health fats. If you're making a salad, boil an egg to go with it and chuck in some walnuts. You get the idea.

Why lunch is important to getting lean

Leaving long gaps between meals is a bad idea because it destabilises blood sugar. There may be some diets that say that fasting is actually good for you (5:2) but in my experience of working with hundreds of clients one to one, I would say that skipping meals causes over-eating at the next one. You are so starving that you literally vacuum up everything you can see in the fridge.

What we also know is that starvation sets off a hormonal cascade that raises the level of a stress hormone called cortisol. This is associated with the laying down of fat in your mid section. So that muffin top can actually be a cortisol belly.

The answer is to space your meals evenly through the day to spread your calorie load and even out mood and energy. Brown bagging is especially useful because it allows you to a) have food available when you need it whether you're near a store or café or not, and b) have the right food available so you're not tempted by a slice of pizza or chocolate bar.

When lunch isn't helping

What are the typical take-out lunches?

Sandwiches, sushi, pasta salad, baked potatoes …

All of these are high in sugar and in the case of sandwiches, made from wheat.

Now, I am not of the 'all wheat is evil' school of nutrition. A wholewheat wrap or pitta can be a healthy option as part of a balanced meal. But there is no doubt that some people are allergic or have an intolerance to grains containing the protein gluten, highest of all in wheat. This can cause bloating, stomach pains, wind and constipation/diarhoea. It can also lead to water retention which makes you look and feel, um, fat.

So, if you are a sandwich addict, I would urge you to think beyond your current prepacked version and consider trying some of the recipes in this book. If you are still unsure, here is the verdict on sandwiches and other popular lunch options:

Sandwiches

Leaving aside the wheat/gluten issue with the bread, many fillings are high in unhealthy fats due to processed meats (ham or bacon) and greasy mayonnaise. To keep costs down and provide a cheap product, manufacturers tend to increase the bread and decrease the filling (the expensive bit) so leading to a protein/carbs/fats ratio that is high on carbs and fats and low on protein. The balance is wrong;

Sushi

Touted as a super-healthy lunch on account of the raw fish (good for healthy fats) and the fact that the rice is low in fat. However, sushi rice is not only white (bad) it is a pudding style rice (badder) and is also sweetened with sugar (baddest). I have clients who love sushi but what they don't realise is the reason they love it is the great wallop of sugar it is giving them. They might as well sit down to a doughut;

Pasta

A take-out pasta salad, restaurant pasta lunch or even a home made pasta dish reheated from the night before is many people's idea of a filling, cheap lunch. However, pasta is a carb and breaks down into sugar in the body. If you go for pasta with a tomato sauce, you are not balancing this sugar with enough protein to keep you stable. You are liable to suffer from reactive hypoglycaemia mid-afternoon as a result of your pasta sugar rush earlier. This will have you rushing for candy at 3pm; and

Rice and Baked Potatoes

The same problem as pasta, only more so. When they measure the Glycaemic Index of white rice and potato (GI is how quickly a carb food turns into sugar in the body), potato and white rice are right up there with table sugar. They are incredibly high energy foods. Adding a sugary tomato-based sauce or a shedload of grated cheddar cheese compounds the problem. You will feel pretty good for about 40 minutes after eating it, then exhausted later on.

Finally

Don't expect to be perfect. We all have slip-ups. If a cake or a bacon sandwich calls to you, don't tell yourself you're a bad person for succumbing. Just start again at your next meal. Congratulate yourself for your efforts and keep going.

I would be very grateful if you would review this book at the end for me when you are prompted to do so. If you are reading this book on an ereader, you will be prompted to add a review at the end. If you are reading this on PC or tablet, you should get a prompt at the end of this book. If you are reading it in paperback (or listening to this in audio when that format arrives soon!), you can leave a review by visiting the book selling platform where you bought the book. I read all my reviews and your views do matter as I update my books based on reader comment and suggestions.

I would also welcome any suggestions for other subjects you would like covered. You can also reach me by email at hello@threepeaspublishing.com if you head your email FAO Maia Lloyd.

Bonus books

Before we get into the meat of my programme, just to let you know that at the back of this book are two free bonus books to download:

The first is one of my books in this series: Eating Clean But Keep It Lean. It is my book on Sweet Treat foods. In it you will find recipes for desserts: from Chocolate Thins and Berry Frozen Yoghurt to Grilled Pears and Ricotta.

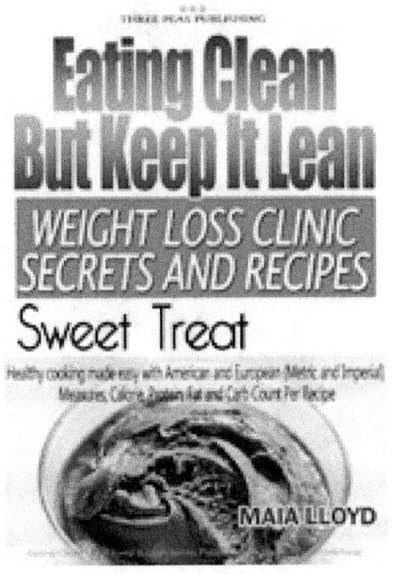

The book also discusses my guidance to my weight loss clients about what makes a dessert Eating Clean But Keep It Lean. Details of how to get this book are at the back of this book with details of all of the books in this Eating Clean But Keep It Lean series.

The other bonus book is from my publishers but it is a good companion to my series. It is called Alcohol Free Drinks and it does what it says on the can, as they say. It probably does a bit more as it is a good mix of celebration drinks, hot toddies, milk shakes, juices and aperitifs. Some of the drinks are higher sugar but they are flagged. The ethos of the book is healthy, natural drinks. No a soda in sight.

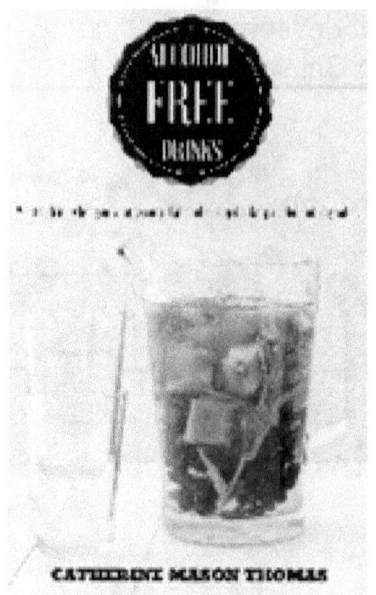

Now on to Chapter 1 and the recipes.

CHAPTER 1
SANDWICHES

Most store-bought sandwiches start with really horrible bread – white and pasty or brown and loaded with added sugars (called malting on the label). You will do so much better if you make your own. Below are some recipes for home-made bread.

However, if you don't have the time or run out, you can still be Eating Clean But Keep It Lean by buying a rye or spelt (a traditional form of wheat that is more easily digested) loaf and using that. Other good loaves are made from other grains like amaranth, buckwheat or quinoa. Sourdough is usually a wheat bread, but again it is much easier to digest and so healthier than mass produced bread.

If you fear that once you make a loaf of any sort of bread you will just go crazy and eat every last crumb, slice it and put it in the freezer straightaway. This portion controls it as well as keeping it fresh.

Spelt and Seed Loaf

A lovely, nutty flavour and firm texture.

Makes: 1 loaf of 10 slices

Preparation: 10 minutes

Cooking: 2 ½ hours to prove, 35 minutes to cook

Ingredients

500g/ 1 lb 2 oz/3 ½ cups spelt flour

300ml/10 fl oz/ ½ pint/1 ¼ cups warm water

2 tablespoons/15ml/1/2 oz agave syrup

1 sachet (7g) dried yeast

2 tablespoons/30g/1 ¼ oz sunflower seeds

2 tablespoons/30g/1 ¼ oz sesame seeds

2 teaspoons/10 g/1/4 oz salt

Olive oil cooking spray

Method

Add the yeast and agave to the water and leave to stand for 10 minutes till frothy. In another bowl, mid the flour, salt and seeds together, make a well in the centre and pour in the yeast mixture. Use your hands to combine the ingredients to a smooth, non sticky dough. Knead for 5 minutes, put back in the bowl, cover with cling film and leave in a warm place for 1 hour till it has doubled in size.

Turn out onto a floured work surface, knead for 3 minutes, put back in the bowl, cover with cling film and leave to rise again for 1 ½ hours.

Preheat the oven to 190/gas mark 5. Turn the dough out onto of the bowl and onto a baking try than has been spritzed with cooking spray. Slash the top of the loaf with a knife and put in the oven to bake for 30 – 35 minutes until it sounds hollow when you knock the bottom. Cut into 10 slices.

Nutritional Content
Makes: 1 loaf of 10 slices
P/slice

Calories 154

Protein 5g

Carbohydrates 4g

Fat 1g

No Knead Buckwheat Bread

This is a quick to make gluten-free bread.

Makes: 1 loaf of 15 slices

Preparation:1 hour 10 minutes to rise

Cooking: 30 minutes

Gluten free

Ingredients

500g/1lb 2 oz/4 cups buckwheat flour or buckwheat groats ground to a powder in a food processor

350ml/11 ½ fl oz/1 ½ cups warm water

1 sachet (7g) dried yeast

2 teaspoons/ 10g/ ¼ oz Stevia based sweetener

2 tablespoons/ 30ml/1 ½ fl oz olive oil

1 teaspoon/ 5g/ ¼ oz salt

1 teaspoon/5ml/1/4 fl oz vinegar

2 eggs

Olive oil cooking spray

Method

Add the yeast and Stevia to the water and leave to stand for 10 minutes. In another bowl, beat the eggs and oil together till frothy. Put the flour and salt in another bowl, make a well in the centre and add the egg mixture, vinegar and yeast mixture. Stir together until you have a wet mixture, more of a very thick batter than a dough. Pour the batter into a loaf tin that has been spritzed with cooking spray. Cover with cling film that has also been spritzed with cooking spray and leave in a warm place for 30 minutes - 1 hour to rise (you want a lift, but if you let it rise too much it will collapse in the oven).

Preheat the oven to 190/gas mark 5. Remove the cling film and bake the bread for 25 – 30 minutes till a skewer comes out clean. Allow to cool and cut into 15 slices

Nutritional content

Makes: 1 loaf of 15 slices

P/slice

Calories 149

Protein 6g

Carbohydrates 23g

Fat 3g

Chickpea and Rosemary Bread

This sounds very odd but it makes a really savoury fragrant loaf. You can also use this recipe to make rolls to have with soup any time. Chickpeas are great at balancing your hormones so good if you get skin break outs or if you are stressed and therefore likely to be producing too much cortisol.

It freezes well.

Makes: 1 loaf of 15 slices

Preparation: 2 hours 20 minutes

Cooking: 30 minutes

Ingredients

400g/14 oz/2 cups canned chickpeas, drained, rinsed and skins removed

500g/1 lb 2 oz/3 ½ cups wholemeal flour, plus extra for kneading

7g sachet yeast

1 teaspoon/ 3g dried rosemary

Zest and juice of ½ lemon

250ml/8 fl oz/1 cup warm water

Olive oil cooking spray

Method

Put the chickpeas in a food processor and process to a rough crumb. Pour into a bowl and add the flour, yeast, rosemary and lemon zest and juice and stir together.. Gradually add enough of the water until you get a soft dough. Turn out onto a floured work surface and knead for 10 minutes. Put back in the bowl, cover with cling film and leave in a wam place for 2 hours till it has doubled in size.

Preheat the oven to 220/gas mark 7. Remove the dough from the bowl and knead again for 1 minute. Put into a loaf tin you have spritzed with cooking spray. Place in the oven and cook for 30 minutes till a skewer comes out clean. Allow to cool and cut into 12 thin slices.

Nutritional Content
Makes: 1 loaf of 15 slices
P/slice

Calories 138

Protein 6g

Carbohydrates 6g

Fat 1g

Wholewheat Pitta Breads

Who would have thought that making pitta breads could be so simple. Still, why bother when you can get them from the shop? Because the shop bought versions have a lot salt, the flour is not particularly good for your blood sugar as it is milled very fine so it acts like a white flour, plus fat is added to give the pittas shelf life.

You can keep these pittas until you need them by freezing them.

Because of the rise time, this is a bread that you treat like installing software, do a bit, come back to it, do a bit more.

Makes: 6 pitta breads

Preparation: 2 hours 10 minutes to prove

Cooking: 12 minutes

Ingredients

500g/ 1lb 2 oz/3 ½ cups wholewheat flour, plus extra for dusting

1 tablespoon/15ml olive oil

1 sachet (7g) dried yeast

1 teaspoon/5g salt

300ml/10 fl oz/1/2 pint/1 ¼ cups warm water

Olive oil cooking spray

Method

Put all the dry ingredients except the spray oil in a bowl, gradually adding the water and mixing with your hands to get a smooth dough. Turn out onto a floured work surface and knead for 5 – 10 minutes. Put back into the bowl, cover with cling film and leave to rise for 1 – 2 hours till it has doubled in size.

Preheat the oven to 250/gas mark 9 and place a clean baking sheet in the middle to heat up. Turn out the dough and knead for 1 minute. Divide it into 6 equal sized balls and flatten to 3 – 5mm thick . Using oven gloves, remove the tray from the oven, dust with flour and place the dough discs on it, leaving space between (you may have to do 2 batches). Bake for 5 – 10 minutes will they have puffed up and are starting to go golden. Allow to cool then split to fill.

Nutritional Content

Makes 6 pitta breads

p/pitta

Calories 290

Protein 10g

Carbohydrates 5g

Fat 4g

Brown Rice Wraps

This is a good recipe to get used to baking with brown rice flour. Rice is of course gluten free so if you have a gluten intolerance and miss bread, this is great for you.

For the rest of us, brown rice flour is also a way to ring the changes and break the over reliance our western diet has on wheat. Plus, because there is no gluten, there is no kneeding or proving for this loaf as no rising so these wraps are quick to make.

This method is very similar to making Indian chapatis, so you can also serve these folded into quarter shapes with a curry for a shared Indian supper.

Makes: 6 wraps

Preparation: 25 minutes

Cooking: 15 minutes

Gluten free

Ingredients

200g/7oz/1 1/3 cup brown rice flour

320ml/10 ½ fl oz/1 1/3 cups water

1 1/2/ tablespoons/20ml olive oil

Pinch of salt

Olive oil cooking spray

Method

Mix all the ingredients except the cooking spray together to form a smooth batter and leave to stand for 20-25 minutes. Spritz a non-stick frying pan with cooking spray and heat. Pour in 2 – 3 tablespoons of the batter and smooth it out to form a pancake. Cook on a medium heat until bubbles form then flip over to cook the other side. Turn out onto a plate and repeat till you have used up all the batter.

Nutritional Content

Makes 6 wraps

P/wrap

Calories 159

Protein 2g

Carbohydrates 2g

Fat 4g

Sandwich Fillings

So, what do you put in your sandwiches? The important thing is to think about balance and ratio. I talked in the introduction to these recipes about the two principles which drive fat loss: blood sugar control and nutrient balance and timing.

In terms of nutrient balance, you want the right rato of macronutrients (carbs, protein and fats). This means making sure you have as much of the filling as you have bread. If your filling is meagre and your bread sliced like house bricks, your sandwiches immediately become too carby, disrupting blood sugar and hormone balance.

You need to add protein and healthy fats to your sandwich to balance the carbs, so some lean chicken or tofu, maybe salmon or avocado for good oils. Plus, don't forget your greens. Adding an handful of nmixed leaves bulks up the sandwiche for very few calories and increases the nutrient content.

Herbs are even better. Ounce for ounce, herbs and spices have a far greater nutrient density than other vegetables. So a pinch of chopped parsley or cayenne packs a really big nutritional punch.

Cottage Cheese and Walnut Slaw

I know, I hate cottage cheese too! But, in this recipe, the best of cottage cheese is used, its creamy consistency. You get the crunch from the beansprouts, walnuts and the onions, the punch from the onions and extra punch, if you opt for it, from the cayenne or paprika.

This is a really nice filling, particulary for the pitta bread, the wrap or the buckwheat bread.

I would make this as near to eating as possible. So if you are brown bagging it, I would make it up in the morning for that day.

Bean sprouts will keep in the fridge for 3 or 4 days. The cottage cheese and spinach for at least a week.

Makes 2 servings

Preparation: 10 minutes

Cooking: none

Vegetarian

Ingredients

1 carrot 75g/3 oz grated

30g/1 ¼ oz beansprouts

1/4 red onion/50g/2 oz, chopped

100g/3 ½ oz cottage cheese

10g/1/4 oz chopped walnuts

1 teaspoon/ 5g sesame seeds

Handful baby spinach leaves

Pinch of cayenne or smoke paprika (optional)

Method

Mix together all the ingredients except the spinach. Lay the spinach on 1 piece of bread, top with the filling and cover with more spinach and the other slice of bread

Nutritional Content

Makes: 2 servings

P/serving

Calories 83

Protein 8g

Carbohydrates 6g

Fat 5g.

Spiced Egg Salad

Eggs: the body builder's favourite. They would eat them plain but this is a far more interesting way to get your protein with a dose of folic acid. The curry powder includes lots of micro nutrients from the spices, the red peppers has phyto nutrients from the red colour.

I put this with the wraps or the seed bread but it will go with any of the bread because it has depth from the curry flavour.

The constituent parts keep perfectly well in the fridge. Boiled eggs can be done ahead of time and will keep for up to five days in the fridge. If you do boil aggs ahead, make sure you keep them differently to your raw eggs so you know which to pick. Otherwise, you are going to be breaking eggs like Ruissian roulette trying to find the cooked ones.

Makes: 2 servings

Preparation: 10 minutes

Cooking: none

Vegetarian

Ingredients

1 hard boiled egg, chopped

2 tablespoons/30ml 0% fat Greek yoghurt

1/2 red pepper, deseeded and chopped

½ teaspoon curry powder

Pinch of salt

4 lettuce leaves

Method

Stir the curry powder and salt into the yoghurt then coat the pepper and egg. Put a lettuce leaf on two slices of bread. Divide the egg mixture between the two, top with another lettuce leaf and another slice of bread.

Nutritional Content

Makes 2 servings

P/serving

Calories 78

Protein 3g

Carbohydrate 2g

Fat 7g

Turkey Cranberry

This recipe also works with turkey or chicken. In either case, left overs from your own cooked meat is best but do what you can and if it is shop bought, this is still a far better sandiwch than you can buy ready made.

Instead of cranberries, you can also use goji berries for extra vitamins and minerals.

This filing goes particularly well with the chickpea and rosemary bread.

This will keep in the fridge for 2-3 days.

Makes: 2 servings

Preparation: 5 minutes

Cooking: none

Ingredients

100g cooked turkey breast, chopped

1 tablespoon/ 10g dried canberries

2 tablespoons/ 30ml/1 fl oz 0% fat Greek yoghurt

50g/1 ¾ oz red onion, finely chopped

Handful of lambs lettuce

Method

Stir all the ingredients together except the lettuce, then place some lettuce on top of two slices of bread. Divide the filling between them and top with more lettuce and another slice of bread.

Nutritional content

Makes 2 servings

P/serving

Calories 112

Protein 17g

Carbohydrates 6g

Fat 2g

Marakesh Chicken Salad

This filling has a definite North African feel and is far more interesting than most of the sandwiches you can buy. As with the turkey cranberry filling, use left over meat if you have it. Otherwise, shop bought meat will do. If you are buying shop bought chicken, if you have a choice, go for the roast, whole breast rather than the slices as they often have added sugar.

Makes: 2 servings

Preparation: 10 minutes

Cooking: none

Ingredients

4 tablespoons/60ml/2 ½ fl oz/1/4 cup Greek 0% fat yoghurt

1 teaspoon/5ml/1/4 fl oz agave syrup

Pinch each dried cumin, cinnamon, cayenne and salt

Sqeeze of lemon juice

100g cooked chicken breast, shredded

1 carrot/25g/1 oz, peeled and grated

1 date, pitted and chopped

Method

Mix together the yoghurt, agave syrup, lemon juice and spices. Then add the chicken, carrot and dates.

Nutritional Content

Makes 2 servings

Calories 153

Protein 18g

Carbohydrates 16g

Fat 2g

Tuna With A Kick

Tuna and cottage cheese gives you the creamy consistency but it can be very bland, at least for my tastes. So I add chilli.

You can also add a couple of black or green olives chopped or some anchovy essence (it comes in a bottle. The brand I use is Geo Watkins Anchovy Sauce, or you can use a single anchovy from a jar patted dry of oil and mashed up. If you are using anchovies from a jar, pick one out with a toothpick so the rest stay in the oil and you do not waste the jar. These twists dial up the flavours a bit.

This will keep in the fridge for 3-4 days.

Makes: 2 servings

Preparation: 10 minutes plus 30 minutes to chill

Cooking: none

Ingredients

60ml/2 ¼ fl oz/1/4 cup low fat cottage cheese

½ teaspoon chilli flakes

150g/ 5oz canned tuna in spring water, drained

Squeeze of lemon juice

1 stick of celery/30g/1 ¼ oz, chopped

Salt and pepper

Bunch of watercress

Method

Put the cottage cheese, chilli, tuna and lemon juice in a food processor and process till smooth. Pour into a bowl and add the celery, salt and pepper. Chill to firm up. Place watercress on two slices of bread. Divide the filling between them and top with more watercress and another slice of bread.

Nutritional Content

Makes 2 servings

P/serving

Calories 98

Protein 20g

Carbohydrates trace

Fat trace

Updated Prawn Cocktail with Avocado

This is my king of sandwich fillings. Avocado with prawns and chilli is just the best. I like this filling on the seed bread or the buckwheat bread.

Makes: 2 servings

Preparation: 5 minutes

Cooking: none

Ingredients

1 tablespoon/15ml cold-pressed extra virgin olive oil

1 teaspoon/5ml lemon juice

Salt and pepper.

100g/3 oz cooked, peeled prawns

½ avocado 40g/1 ½ oz, sliced thinly

½ fennel bulb 110g/3 ¾ oz, sliced very thinly

2 spring onions, chopped

Handful of wild rocket

A pinch of chilli powder if you like it.

Method

Mix together the oil, lemon juice, salt and pepper, then gently coat the prawns and fennel with this. Place some rocket on two slices of bread. Divide the filling and pile on top of rocket. Top with avocado and sprinkle on the spring onions. Top with more rocket and another slice of bread.

Nutritional Content

Makes 2 servings

P/serving

Calories 115

Protein 8g

Carbohydrates 4g

Fat 6g.

Asian Crayfish and Cucumber

Another good prawn recipe. I think any sandwich filling with prawns is automatically in another league. It does not feel like you are denying yourself, if anything, quite the opposite.

Makes: 2 servings

Preparation: 5 minutes

Cooking: none

Ingredients

150g/5 oz peeled, cooked prawns

4 tablespoons/ 60ml/1/4 cup 0% fat Greek yoghurt

¼ teaspoon thai curry paste

Squeeze of lemon juice

1 tablespoon/10g chopped coriander

½ cucumber 200g/7 oz sliced

8 butter lettuce leaves

Method

Stir the curry paste into the yoghurt and then pour over the prawns and cucumber, add the lemon juice and fresh coriander. Put 2 lettuce leaves on two slices of bread and divide the filling between them. Top with two more lettuce leaves each and a slice of bread each.

Nutritional Content

Makes 2 servings

P/serving

Calories 85

Protein 15g

Carbohydrate 3g

Fat 1g

CHAPTER 2
LUNCHPOTS

Lunchpots are new on the packed lunch scene. Now that most offices have microwaves they allow you to have a hot lunch while still being chained to your desk! Great! If you're at home they are undeniably quick and easy. The problem is so many of them are total garbage. White rice or pasta topped with a highly processed sauce... Book yourself in for your heart bypass now.

So, I decided to try to come up with some ideas for Eating Clean But Keep It Lean lunch pots. You need to get yourself a pot with a tight-fitting lid – no-one wants a handbag full of tomato sauce. You can also now buy insulated plastic pots or bowls with screw lids so even if you do not have a microwave at work, you can have a hot meal as lunchtime as these pots or bowls keep the food warm for hours.

My recipes are really easy to make so give them a go.

Middle Eastern Chickpea, Coconut and Spinach Lunch Pot

I find that coconut milk is really satisfying in a stew or gravy. One tip with coconut milk, rather han buying the reduced fat one, but the normal one and dilute it with water 1:1. The ginger in this is also very warming and ginger settles your stomach so if you are not feeling on top form, this is a good meal to help you get back on top form.

Makes: 2 servings

Preparation: 10 minutes

Cooking: 25 minutes

Vegetarian

Ingredients

Olive oil cooking spray

1/2 small onion 75g/2 1/2oz

2 cloves garlic, crushed

1/2 tablespoon/7g grated ginger

1 tablespoon/15ml/1/2 fl oz tomato paste

Zest and juice of 1/2 lemon

Pinch chilli flakes

400g/14 oz/2 cups canned chickpeas, drained

300g baby spinach leaves

200g/7oz/1 cup reduced fat coconut milk

Pinch ground ginger

1/2 teaspoon/2.5g Stevia-based sweetener

Method

Spritz a saucepan with spray oil and gently fry the onion for 5 minutes till softened, then add the garlic, ginger, tomato paste, lemon zest and chilli flakes and fry for 3 minutes, stirring. Add some water if it starts to stick. Add the chick peas and cook for 3 minutes, coating them in the mixture, then add the spinach, reserving a little to top the pots. Add it a bit at time, wilting it in the pan.When all the spinach has wilted, pour in the coconut milk, ginger and Stevia . Simmer gently for 10 minutes, add the lemon juice and allow to cool. Pour into pots and top with the reserved fresh spinach leaves.

Nutritional Content

Makes 2 servings

Calories 342

Protein 15g

Carbohydrates 38g

Fat 11g

<u>Dhal with Broccoli Lunch Pot</u>

This feels like comfort food. Turmeric in particular is a fantastic, health supporting spice. Broccoli is also the king of vegetables for supporting detoxification in your liver. So, if you have over indulged or been drinking, this is an excellent pick me up lunch.

The dhal can be made in big batches and frozen. The easiest way to freeze this would be to use the ice cube trays that people use to freeze baby food – the compartments are bigger than conventional ice cube trays. Freeze it like that and then pop the ice cubes onto a freezer bag, ready to use.

Makes: 2 servings

Preparation: 10 minutes

Cooking: 30 minutes

<u>Ingredients</u>

150g/5 oz/1/2 cup dried red lentils

1 teaspoon/5g turmeric

1 tablespoon 15g/1/4 oz tamarind paste

Pinch of salt

120ml/4 fl oz/1/2 cup water

Olive oil cooking spray

1 onion/200g/7 oz, chopped finely

1 cloves garlic, crushed

3cm piece of ginger, peeled and grated

1 teaspoons/5g curry powder

250g/9 oz broccoli, broken into small florets, stem discarded

Method

Put the lentils, turmeric, tamarind, salt and water in a saucepan. Bring up to the boil, put a lid on and simmer for 15 minutes until the lentils are soft. Meanwhile spritz a non-stick frying pan with spray oil and gently fry the onion for 5 minutes, till soft. Add the garlic, and ginger and cook for a further 2 minutes. If it starts to stick, add a splash of water. Stir in the curry powder and cook for 2 minutes, pour in the lentils and cook for 10 minutes. Boil or steam the broccoli until tender, rinse in cold water and set aside. Pour the dhal into the pots and top with the broccoli.

Nutritional Content

Makes 2 servings

Calories 335

Protein 24g

Carbohydrates 50g

Fat 26g

Sweet and Sour Pork Lunch Pot

Doing a sweet and sour pot was a challenge I set myself because it's such a popular fast food lunch idea. This freezes well but make the rice no more than three days on advance. A note about storing cooked rice. If you do not intend to eat it straight away, cool it down quickly by running cold water over it and then cover it and refridgerate it immediately. The reason is that if you leave rice to cool down slowly, you risk food poisoning.

Makes 2 servings

Preparation: 10 minutes

Cooking: 10 minutes

<u>Ingredients</u>

50 ml water

1 tablespoon/15g/1/2 oz cornflour

1 tablespoon/15g/1/2 oz tomato paste

1 teaspoon/5g soy sauce

1 teaspoon/5g Stevia-based sweetener

40ml/1 ¾ oz/1/4cup rice wine vinegar

Spray olive oil

200g/7 oz lean pork, but into small pieces

1/2 red and 1/2 green pepper 175g//6oz, deseeded and chopped

300g/11 oz/1 ½ cups cooked wholemeal brown rice

<u>Method</u>

Mix the water and cornflour until smooth. Then add the soy, tomato puree, Stevia and vinegar. Spritz a wok with cooking spray and fry the pork for 2 – 3 minutes. Lift out and set aside. Add the peppers and and fry for 2 – 3 minutes. If they start to stick add a splash of water. Pour in the cornflour mixture and cook for 2 – 3 minutes, then put the pork back in for 1 minute. Turn off the heat and allow to cool. Put the rice at the bottom of each pot, top with the pork mixture.

Nutritional Content

Makes 2 servings

P/serving

Calories 342

Protein 28g

Carbohydrates 44g

Fat 6g

Paella Lunch Pot

This recipe uses quinoa in place of rice for the paella. Quinoa is much higher in protein.

This will keep in the fridge covered for two days.

Makes: 2 servings

Preparation: 10 minutes

Cooking: 25 minutes

Ingredients

Zest and juice of ½ lemon

2 cloves garlic, crushed

1 teaspoon/5g smoked paprika

Pinch of salt

200g/7oz fresh prawns,peeled and deveined

Olive oil cooking spray

1 onion 200g/7oz, chopped

125g/4oz/ 1 cup quinoa

300g/11oz cauliflower, chopped

400ml water

50g/3oz frozen peas

1 tablespoon/10g/1/4 oz fresh, chopped parsley

Method

Combine the garlic, lemon juice, paprika and salt in a bowl and add the prawns, coating them. Set aside. Spritz a non-stick pan with cooking spray and fry the onion for 5 minutes till soft. Add the quinoa, turmeric and water, bring to the boil, then reduce to a simmmer. Put a lid on and cook for 10 – 15 minutes. Meanwhile put the cauliflower in the food processor and process to a rice consistency.

5 minutes before the end of the quinoa's cooking time, add the cauliflower and the peas, bring back up the boil and put the lid back on. When the quinoa is cooked, turn off theheat and set aside. Spritz a non stick pan with cooking spray and fry the prawns for 1 – 2 minutes on each side till no longer pink. Allow everything to cool then put the quinoa in the bottom of the pots, add the prawns and sprinkle with parsley.

Nutritional Content

Makes 2 servings

P/serving

Calories 395

Protein 77g

Carbohydrates 52g

Fat 12g

Provencal Tuna Ratatouille Lunchpot

You can eat this hot or cold. Be sure to simmer the vegatables slowly to avoid burning them and giving the sauce a bitter taste.

Makes 2 servings

Ingredients

Olive oil cooking spray

1/2 onion 100g/3 ½ oz, chopped

1 red pepper/175g/6oz deseeded and chopped

1 clove garlic, crushed

1 sprig rosemary

1/2 aubergine 125g/4oz, diced

1 courgette/150g/5oz, diced

400g/14oz/2 cups canned chopped tomatoes

1 teaspoon balsamic vinegar

175g/6oz canned tuna steak in spring water

Handful of fresh basil leaves.

195g/70z/1 cup cooked wholemeal rice

Method

Spritz a non-stick saucepan with spray oil and fry the onion and pepper for 5 minutes, then add the garlic and cook for another 1 minute. If it starts to stick, add a splash of water. Add the vegetables and tomatoes. Bring up to the boil then turn down to a simmer, leaving the lid off cook for 20 minutes till the vegetables are cooked and the sauce has reduced. Stir in the vinegar. Allow to cool. Put the rice at the bottom of the pots, followed by the ratatouille and top each with half the tuna and fresh basil leaves

Nutritional Content

Makes 2 servings

P/serving

Calories 292

Protein 39g

Carbohydrate 35g

Fat 5g

CONCLUSION

So there we are, sandwiches and pots that are balanced and gentle on your blood sugar.

The legal bit is next and then I have some concluding thoughts about weight loss, details of how to download my free, bonus books and also news of the rest of my series: **Eating Clean But Keep It Lean**.

I hope that you have been inspired to take control of your lunches and make them part of your nutritional approach, not a cul de sac that you go down each lunch time, only to emerge at dinner and try to get yourself back on track.

Brown bagging your lunch means no more standing in a gas station, corner shop or deli faced by a wall of high fat, high sugar foods and unable to decide which one to assault your body with. Instead, you'll be able to be consistent in your healthy food choices. This way of eating is for the long haul, so finding a way to be healthy every day is key.

If you'd like some more lunch ideas, why not check out the other lunch recipe book in this series – Soups and Salad. Or get inspired by my books on Breakfast, Dinners and Snacks (details at the end of this book).

I also look at all my reviews and I would be really grateful if you would post a review of this book. You will be prompted at the end of this book to post a star rating and a review. Please let me know what you thought of it.

Finally, well done on choosing to eat the best you can for health and leanness. You will never regret looking after your health and body. My clients never do.

If you enjoyed this book, this is part of a whole series I have written to publish my recipes from my weight loss clinics. One of these books, the Sweet Treat recipe book, is free as part of my bonus books (see below), the others are my nutritional plans focussed on real food eaten everyday and are available from Amazon.

Each book has lots of recipes from my clinics, ones that have worked with my clients to help them lose weight. The introduction to each book also tells a little of the story of my approach at my clinics so you understand what foods and recipes are best for weight loss.

You can find the complete series, book by book, at Amazon and they are also listed below. Get the set or start off with a couple of books to inspire you and inform you about the Eating Clean But Keep it Lean approach to particular meals, say Dinner and Brown Bag Lunches, for example.

If you have comments or questions, you can also get in contact with me by emailing me at hello@threepeaspublishing.com

Here is the complete series. You can buy single books or the whole series.

Just search "Maia Lloyd Author Page" on Amazon

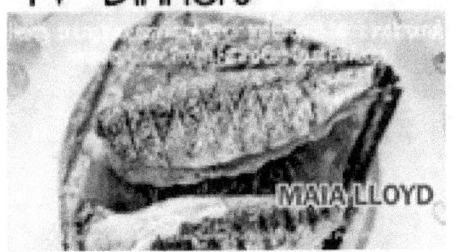

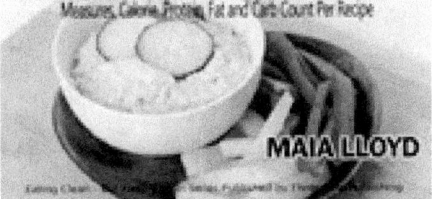

THREE PEAS PUBLISHING

Eating Clean But Keep It Lean

WEIGHT LOSS CLINIC SECRETS AND RECIPES

Soups & Salads

Healthy cooking made easy with American and European (Metric and Imperial) Measures, Calorie, Protein, Fat and Carb Count Per Recipe

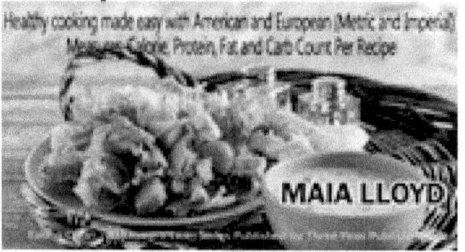

MAIA LLOYD

THREE PEAS PUBLISHING

Eating Clean But Keep It Lean

WEIGHT LOSS CLINIC SECRETS AND RECIPES

Brown Bag Lunches

Healthy cooking made easy with American and European (Metric and Imperial) Measures, Calorie, Protein, Fat and Carb Count Per Recipe

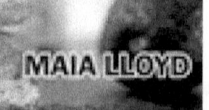

MAIA LLOYD

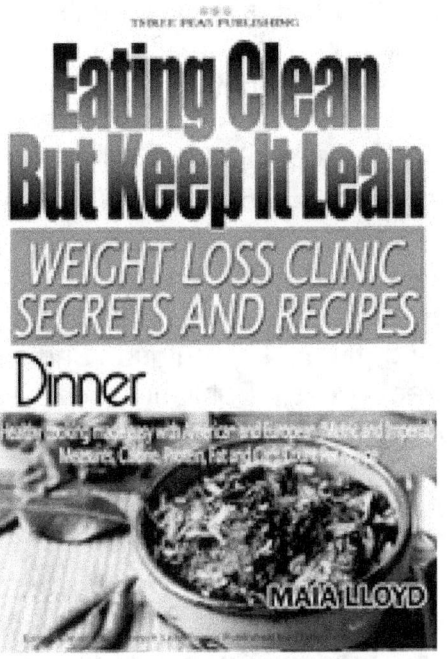

Bonus books

The first is one of my books in this series: Eating Clean But Keep It Lean. It is my book on Sweet Treat foods. In it you will find recipes for desserts: from Chocolate Thins and Berry Frozen Yoghurt to Grilled Pears and Ricotta.

The book also discusses my guidance to my weight loss clients about what makes a dessert Eating Clean But Keep It Lean.

You can download this at:
www.threepeaspublishing.com/eatingcleanbutkeepitleanswe ettreat

The other bonus book is from my publishers but it is a good companion to my series. It is called Alcohol Free Drinks and it does what it says on the can, as they say. It probably does a bit more as it is a good mix of celebration drinks, hot toddies, milk shakes, juices and aperitifs. There are a few higher sugar drinks but they are flagged. The rest are very healthy and not a soda in sight.

You can download this at:
www.threepeaspublishing.com/alcoholfreedrinks

If you are interested in nutrition, fitness and wellness, you can subscribe to news, offers and How To videos on nutrition (including my books), nutrition and resilience via my publisher, Three Peas Publishing. To subscribe, go to www.threepeaspublishing.com. Three Peas Media also has a YouTube Channel "Three Peas Media" which provides videos on fitness and nutrition and resilience.

Finally, I would be very grateful if you would review this book for me when you are prompted to do so if you are reading this book on an ereader, or by visiting the book selling platform if you are reading this in paperback. I read all my reviews and I would also welcome and suggestions for other subjects you would like covered. You can also reach me by email at hello@threepeaspublishing.com if you head your email FAO Maia Lloyd.

Good luck and value your health.

With best wishes

Maia Lloyd

Good luck.

Maia Lloyd

www.ingramcontent.com/pod-product-compliance
Lightning Source LLC
Chambersburg PA
CBHW071132280526
45787CB00003B/1257